THE AT-HOME GYM SERIES

WEIGHT MACHINES

WEIGHT MACHINES

THE WEIGHT MACHINES
TRAINING PROGRAM
AND
BUYER'S GUIDE

by Judith Zimmer

Technical consultant: Andrew Irsay
Introduction by
Gabe Mirkin, M.D.,
and Mona Shangold, M.D.

VILLARD BOOKS
New York   1985

The instructions and advice in this book are in no way intended as a substitute for medical counseling. We advise anyone to consult with a doctor before beginning this or any other exercise program.

JUDITH ZIMMER is a writer whose work has appeared in *Mademoiselle, Esquire, Psychology Today, Health,* and *The New York Daily News.* She has written a forthcoming book on endurance sports.

ANDREW IRSAY is an Olympic weight trainer and a world-class champion himself. He is now retired from competition and coaches amateurs and professionals on a one-to-one basis.

Photographs by Ken Levinson

Information on pages 6 and 7 from Helane Royce, *Sportshape* (New York: Priam Books/Arbor House, 1983). Reprinted by permission.

Gym facilities courtesy of Christian Dior Lingerie and Chevette.

Produced by the Miller Press

Library of Congress Catalog Card Number: 84-40599

ISBN: 0-394-72974-9

Manufactured in the United States of America

9 8 7 6 5 4 3 2

First Edition

CONTENTS

There are numerous basic components to total fitness; among them are strength, cardiovascular fitness, speed, coordination, and muscle flexibility. Any sensible, well-thought-out exercise program will include different types of activities, each of which will help promote the development of one or more of the components of total fitness.

The At-Home Gym Series* presents a wide range of exercises that will help you reach your goal of total fitness. Each book in the series covers a specific activity (rowing, stationary cycling, free-weight training, to name a few), detailing the special exercises and training routines to follow for each. By combining the instructions contained in each book in the series, *you can design your own total-fitness program* . . . you can apply the principles of total fitness and of specific training as you *tailor your exercise program to* particular goals.

Before you embark on your total-fitness program, it is important to know something of the physiology of exercise.

Exercises can be divided into two categories: *anaerobic exercises,* which focus on your heart's ability to pump oxygen to the muscles through the bloodstream.

Strength is achieved through short bursts of exercise lasting 30 to 50 seconds and performed against resistance. These are the *anaerobic exercises,* and they include weight lifting, working out on Universal or Nautilus-type weight machines, and sprinting.

The way to make a muscle stronger is to stretch that muscle while it contracts. In weight lifting, your muscles actually stretch before the weight starts to move. The first time that you lift a weight, you use only a few of your muscle fibers. But with each successive lift, you use more fibers until the muscle eventually begins to accumulate breakdown

---

*For other books in this series, see last page of this book.—ED.

products of metabolism and becomes acidic. Since muscle acidity restricts the number of fibers that can contract, you lose the effectiveness of such strengthening exercises after the brief initial burst—10 to 12 repetitions for weight lifters or 100 to 250 yards for sprinters.

Cardiovascular fitness or endurance is achieved through continuous moderate exercise over periods of no less than 10 minutes. These are the *aerobic exercises*, and they include cycling, rowing, swimming, jogging, dancing, jumping rope, and brisk walking.

In cardiovascular or endurance activities, the heart muscle itself is the one receiving the workout. The body's muscles demand a continuous, elevated supply of oxygen during a workout. Your heart is like a balloon that relaxes to fill with blood and then squeezes this blood from its chambers to the rest of your body. The more blood you have inside your heart when the muscle contracts, the greater the resistance the heart muscle encounters and the stronger it becomes.

Always remember that you must engage in *specific* training activities in order to become proficient in *each area* of fitness. For example, you cannot train for strength at the same time you train for cardiovascular fitness. When you engage in several different forms of specific training, however, you will be well on your way to total fitness.

By acquainting yourself with the basic principles of fitness and by following the guidelines set forth in the various books in The At-Home Gym Series, you can set up and develop your own exercise program without joining a costly health club and without venturing outdoors in brutal summer heat or numbing winter cold. Don't forget to supplement your exercises with the appropriate warm-up and cooldown periods, as outlined in The At-Home Gym Series, and to consult your physician before engaging in any new activity or whenever you are injured.

And enjoy your journey down the path to total fitness!

—GABE MIRKIN, M.D.
MONA SHANGOLD, M.D.

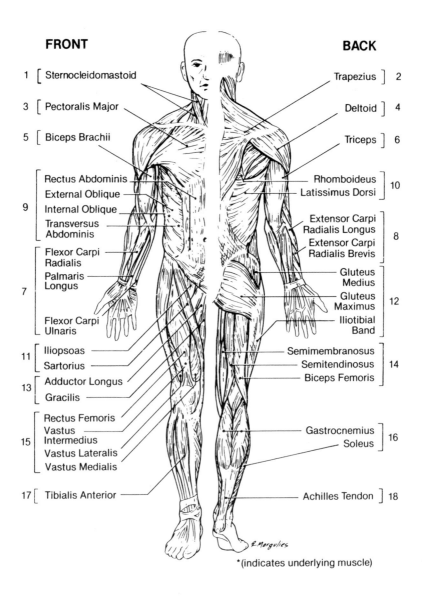

FRONT

1 [Sternocleidomastoid

3 [Pectoralis Major

5 [Biceps Brachii

Rectus Abdominis
External Oblique
9   Internal Oblique
Transversus
Abdominis

Flexor Carpi
Radialis
Palmaris
7   Longus

Flexor Carpi
Ulnaris

11 [Iliopsoas
Sartorius

13 [Adductor Longus
Gracilis

Rectus Femoris
Vastus
15 Intermedius
Vastus Lateralis
Vastus Medialis

17 [Tibialis Anterior

BACK

Trapezius] 2

Deltoid] 4

Triceps] 6

Rhomboideus
Latissimus Dorsi] 10

Extensor Carpi
Radialis Longus
Extensor Carpi
Radialis Brevis] 8

Gluteus
Medius
Gluteus
Maximus
Iliotibial
Band] 12

Semimembranosus
Semitendinosus
Biceps Femoris] 14

Gastrocnemius
Soleus] 16

Achilles Tendon] 18

R.Margulies

*(indicates underlying muscle)

6

MUSCLE	ACTION
1 Sternocleidomastoid	Tucks chin and rotates head.
2 Trapezius	Lifts shoulders.
3 Pectoralis Major	Pulls arms forward and across the chest.
4 Deltoid	Lifts arms at a right angle to the trunk; assists arms to move forward or backward.
5 Biceps Brachii	Flexes or bends the elbow joint.
6 Triceps	Extends or straightens the forearm and the elbow joint.
7 Flexor Carpi Radialis, Flexor Carpi Ulnaris and Palmaris Longus	Flexes the wrist downward and to both sides.
8 Extensor Carpi Radialis Longus and Brevis	Extends the wrist.
9 External and Internal Oblique, Rectus Abdominis and Transversus Abdominis	Rotates the trunk. Flattens the abdomen.
10 Rhomboideus Latissimus Dorsi	Downward and backward movement of the arms.
11 Iliopsoas, Sartorius	Lifts the thigh and flexes and rotates the hip.
12 Gluteus Medius, Gluteus Maximus	Controls outward leg motion; powers the hip for movement.
Iliotibial Band	Gives lateral stability to the knee.
13 Adductor Longus	Outward leg motion.
Gracilis	Inward leg motion.
14 Semimembranosus, Semitendinosus, Biceps Femoris	Hamstrings; flex the leg and rotate the knee.
15 Rectus Femoris, Vastus Intermedius, Vastus Lateralis, Vastus Medialis	Quadriceps group; extends the knee and flexes the hip.
16 Gastrocnemius	Working together to raise the heel and extend the foot.
Soleus	Constantly in use for standing, walking, running and jumping.
17 Tibialis Anterior	Flexes the foot; changes direction while running and is most responsible for shin splints.
18 Achilles Tendon	Attaches the calf muscles to the heel (the gastroc-soleus group).

INTRODUCTION TO WEIGHT TRAINING

Building a better body has been an American pastime for decades. In the '30s and '40s, there was "the insult that made a man out of Mac," the well-known cartoon in advertising history in which the skinny boy on the beach gets sand kicked in his face by the big bully. The ad inspired millions of skinny boys to send away for the Charles Atlas home exercise program.

Today, the inspiration to build a fine physique is firmly ingrained in our culture: Few need to be bullied into working out. The fitness boom is so widespread that there are more ways than one to develop a fine, well-toned body—even at home.

Back in the '30s and '40s, there was only one way to build muscles (that is, one way besides the Charles Atlas exercise program) and that was by performing a series of exercises that involved lifting barbells and dumbbells. Free weights, as these mobile weights are called, are still popular and are regarded as the granddaddy of weight training.

In 1957, a new form of weight training was invented, designed to cut down on the time it took to do free-weight exercises. A company called Universal created the first weight-training machine that incorporated the same principles of lifting used in free weights.

Although weight training with machines has been around for decades, it's been only in the past few years that it has gained popularity in health clubs, fitness centers, and home gyms. What once appeared to be an alienating labyrinth of metal jungle gym has been updated, uplifted, and technologically improved to make weight training accessible, inexpensive, convenient, challenging, safe, easy, and fast.

Weight training opens up a whole new world of fitness. It is not designed to give you an aerobic workout, but it will strengthen your muscles. Remember that both cardiovascular fitness and strength-training exercises are components of total fitness. Weight training strengthens (and reduces injury to) muscles that you'll use in aerobic exercise.

Unlike running and swimming, which exercise and strengthen large muscle groups like the legs or back, weight training gives each muscle an individual workout. For example, there are more ways than one to strengthen a weak tennis arm. To supplement on-court training, take that forearm, divide it into biceps and triceps, and work each muscle part. The same goes for a swimmer's stroking arm, a runner's calves, or a gymnast's lower back.

How does weight training work? The principle behind weight training is resistance. You develop muscle strength by lifting, pulling, or pushing against something that resists you: it can be your own weight, gravity, or free weights. Resistance works the muscles in two ways: first, the muscle contracts and shortens. Then, as the weight is brought down, the muscle lengthens. Both parts of the exercise build muscle strength.

Before you get started, we want to open your eyes to the benefits of weight training by clearing up two common misconceptions:

Myth #1

Weight training will make me look unnaturally muscular.
Wrong. Believe it or not, you have control over your own

body. Bodybuilders develop large, bulging muscles because they want them. Chances are, you'll want to define and tone the muscles you already have (especially flabby ones). Whether you go beyond tone and definition is up to you.

Myth #2

Women with muscles lose their femininity.

Wrong. Women are genetically different from men. Your physiological makeup won't allow you to be anything but female! Working out with weights trims flab, firms up curves, and helps you stay in shape. A well-toned, firm, strong female body is not only accepted, but encouraged and desired.

What will weight training do for me?

- **Weight training is not for men—or he-men—only. Everyone looks better when fit. And weight training will contribute to everyone's overall fitness.**
- **Weight training builds muscle strength by concentrating on each muscle group.**
- **Weight training allows you to see the toning and tightening up of the muscles as they happen.**
- **Weight training conditions you for every other sport and helps you reduce the chance of injury, since strong muscles can tolerate a tougher, more stressful workout.**
- **Like any other fitness activity, weight training gives you an energy boost that will help you get through the rest of the day.**
- **Weight training builds muscle and burns fat. So don't be surprised if, after the first month of the program, you step on the scale and find your weight has gone up: muscle weighs more than fat. Don't expect to lose *weight*. Expect to reduce flab and fat. To see any weight loss result, you must combine physical activity with a good, healthy diet. That means eating well-balanced meals and cutting back on sweets and fatty or fried foods.**

Today, high-tech weight machines let us choose how we want to build muscles. There are two main types of weight-training machines for the home gym: the multi-station machine and the Nautilus machine.

The Multi-Station Machines

Multi-station machines are complete workout centers that come in a variety of shapes and sizes. Some are designed with an elegant line and an eye toward storage; they are either free standing or can be mounted on the wall. Others are similar to the fitness centers in commercial gyms and health spas.

The basic components of a multi-station machine are a bench press, a pulldown attachment, and a set of pulleys for additional arm and leg work. There are one or more stacks of weights attached to the machine and a selector pin for easy weight selection.

Nautilus

The first high-tech weight-training machines of their kind, Nautilus equipment is designed to speed up the weight-training workout. Many gyms, health clubs, and spas feature Nautilus—30 separate exercise stations, which work out each muscle group.

Recently, the company has created exercise machines for the home. So far, they offer an abdominal machine and a lower back machine. A biceps/triceps machine, an exercise bike, a multi-station center, and four machines for basic muscle groups will be added to the Nautilus line.

The philosophy behind Nautilus equipment—for both the home and gym—is the same. Unlike other weight-training units, your body becomes part of the machine. You select the weight, sit in a seat or lie back on the machine, strap yourself in, and go. There's only one way to sit or stand in the machine, so there's less chance of error and, because the machine puts your body into position, the workout goes fast. Of course, you still have to perform the exercises properly—Nautilus won't do that for you. But maintaining a correct, safe position in these machines is easier than maintaining it in a multi-station unit.

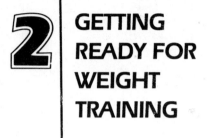

GETTING READY FOR WEIGHT TRAINING

Safety and Form

Because each stack of weights is set into the machine, there is never any worry that a weight will fall on your foot or your head. In that way, weight machines are safer than doing barbell and dumbbell exercises. There are, however, a few danger spots to be aware of:

1. Lift a safe amount of weight.

The amount of weight you lift is important to a safe workout. Be sure you don't lift more weight than you can handle. That can overexert muscles and harm them unnecessarily. It's always better to start out with a low weight and build from that. You'll increase your self-confidence as you increase the weight.

2. Proper form ensures a safe workout.

Even though weight machines are designed for a quick, thorough workout, you can still injure yourself if you perform exercises incorrectly. Resist the temptation to wiggle, jilt, or throw one side of your chest or one arm into the exercise to get that extra push. For example, wiggling under a weight while doing heavy bench pressing can harm your back. Also, you will be exercising one part of your body more than the other.

Proper form is essential to a good workout. Learn to do the exercises correctly. If you are sloppy about performing them, you won't get a good workout at all.

It's always wise to exercise with other people within earshot so that if you do injure yourself, you have help nearby. When you're doing difficult moves—like the bench press and the press behind the neck—it's a good idea to have a spotter, someone to stand at your side while you exercise, to make sure you can handle the weights.

Breathing

Correct breathing is a part of good form. Always inhale just before the exercise and exhale on the effort. It's simply more comfortable to do it that way. If you inhale while lifting a weight, you will be contracting your muscles against inhalation and there won't be enough room for your lungs to expand with air.

Muscle Ache

With any sport, when you work your muscles hard, they feel it. The same goes with weights. Besides learning how to do the exercises correctly, your body will be learning how it feels to work out. When you perform the exercises correctly, you feel it. Your muscles ache. As soon as you stop exercising, they stop hurting. If you are injuring yourself, you'll feel that, too. Instead of a dull ache throughout the working muscle, you'll feel a sharp pain in a joint. Your position is wrong. Stop immediately. Take a few minutes to reassess your position. If the pain goes away immediately, resume the set, using a lighter weight.

Use the feeling in your muscles as an indication of your workout. Some people stop as soon as they feel any discomfort—and you might want to—but don't. That low-level pain means you are working to capacity and your muscles are getting stronger.

What to Expect From Your Body

Don't expect to feel or see results from your training program overnight. Working toward a fit, trim body takes time, discipline, and patience. During the first two weeks of your exercise program, you'll feel a slight ache in your muscles (that will remind you of your workouts) when you climb stairs or lift a heavy package. That muscle discomfort is part of your body's building process: it is getting used to the training. By the third week, you'll start to feel healthy. Just working out regularly will give you that fit, energetic feeling.

We recommend that you continue with this basic weight-training program for 14 to 16 weeks. After that time, your body will be used to the training and you will see the results in your muscle tone. With four months of training under your belt, your muscles will look bigger and you'll begin to feel stronger.

What to wear. **To be safe, always protect your feet by wearing sneakers. Never go barefoot! While you're warming up, wear a sweatsuit. But then strip down to shorts and a T-shirt for the workout. You'll want to see your muscles working.**

Warm-up

Warming up is a must. It loosens your muscles and gets them ready to work. Through practice, you'll discover what works best for you: aerobic conditioning, abdominals or a combination of both. But be sure you don't burn out on the warm-up. You'll want to reserve energy for the machines.

Resting muscle temperature is about 98°F., and muscles are more likely to tear at this temperature. When you exercise at a relaxed pace for a minute or so before the workout, your muscles can warm up to 101°F. or more, at which point they are more pliable and less likely to be injured.

- For the upper body—Do side bends. Then do twists from the waist up, bringing the shoulders around.
- For arms—Do windmills, extending the arms out to the sides. Rotate them in large circles, then smaller ones.
- For aerobic warm-up—Jog in place, jump rope, or use your exercise bicycle for five minutes.

Stretching

Warning: Do not stretch before you warm up—you may wind up pulling a muscle. You stretch to make your muscles more flexible. Every time you exercise, your muscles are injured slightly; when they heal, they shorten. Always warm up before you stretch. Stretching cold muscles is more likely to tear them.

- Stretch: Do two or three stretching exercises, such as toe touches, side bends, and windmills. For legs—In a standing position, cross one leg over the other and touch your toes, keeping the pelvis back. Switch legs. On the floor, sit with your legs extended in front of you and reach for your toes. Next, straddle legs, and again, reach for your toes.

Cool-down

This phase protects you from feeling dizzy after you have completed your workout. When your leg muscles relax, the veins near them fill up with blood. When the muscles contract, they press against the veins near them, squeezing the blood back toward the heart. If you stop exercising suddenly, blood pools in the legs and not enough may be available to reach the brain, in which case you feel dizzy. To prevent this, simply slow down gradually when you work out.

EQUIPMENT FOR ABDOMINAL EXERCISES
Exercise Mat

Abdominal Exercises

Abdominal exercises are a necessary part of every weight session. They round out the workout by strengthening muscles that would otherwise remain untouched. They train you to breathe deeply from the diaphragm and give the final touch to the physique by tightening up the tummy. Like weight-training exercises themselves, doing abdominal exercises hurts. When done correctly, they make your stomach muscles cry out for you to stop. Don't. Try them before or after your workout or in two broken-up sets, one before and one after.

ELBOW-TO-BENT-KNEES
30 reps, 15 to each side

Lie on your back on the floor, knees bent. Place your hands behind your head. Lift your upper body and touch one knee; lie back down. Lift again, alternate elbow to knee.

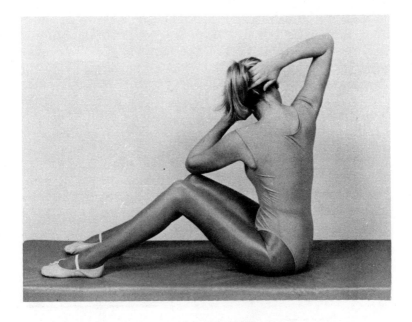

QUARTER-UPS
25 to 30 reps

Lie on your back on the floor, knees bent. Hands behind head. Lift your head and chest, keeping lower back flat on the ground. Your upper abdominals will tighten. Slowly lower chest and head to floor. Repeat.

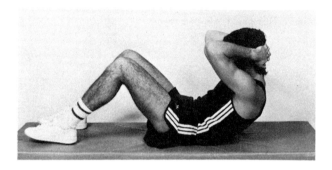

CRUNCHES WITH CROSSED ANKLES
40 reps

Lie on your back, hands behind head. Lift your legs and cross your ankles in the air. Bring both elbows to your knees. Squeeze the stomach muscles and "crunch" them by pressing in with your legs at the same time you raise your elbows. Slowly lower chest and head to floor. Repeat.

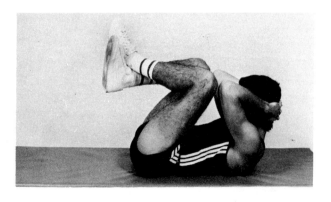

CYCLES
40 reps, 20 to each side

Lie on your back, hands behind head. One leg is bent, the other extended straight. Bring elbow to opposite (bent) knee, always keeping the other leg extended. Your legs will be bicycling.

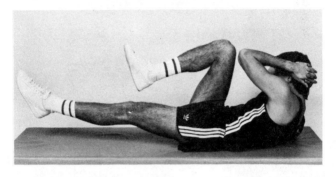

THE WEIGHT-TRAINING PROGRAM

Use these guidelines to establish your weight-training program:

1. Plan to use your machines every other day. Weight training is too strenuous to do daily. If you did work out every day, you wouldn't be giving your muscles the rest and recovery they need between workouts. Building strength is a two-fold process: pushing working muscles to the limit and then giving them a chance to recover.

2. Set aside between 30 minutes and an hour for each workout. On days when you're in a hurry, you can condense and speed up your program. When you do have the time to enjoy your equipment, extend the workout.

3. How much weight should you lift? The range of weight that your machine handles will depend on which one you buy. When purchasing a machine, that's one of the criteria to look for. (See Buyer's Guide to Weight-Training Machines, pp. 42-57.)

Before you establish the pattern of a regular workout, you won't know how much weight you're capable of lifting. Experiment. Start with a small amount and then go on to the next level if that's not hard enough. (See the next chapter for guidelines.)

4. Weight training is done by performing the same movement over and over again in a steady cadence called repetitions, or reps. To get any benefit at all, you must do between 10 and 14 reps of each exercise without stopping. When using a multi-station unit, do the first set of 12 and then rest for about a minute before starting the next set of exercises. The Nautilus home gym machines are different from the multi-station machines and the Nautilus commercial machines. The Nautilus home machines work the abdominals and lower back—muscles that are developed with a lot of repetitions—it is suggested that you do only one set, starting with about 20 to 25 reps and working up to about 40 without stopping.

For your first three workouts, we suggest you do only 10 reps on each machine so your body can get used to the feeling. After the first week, follow the rep guidelines recommended for each exercise.

5. The first eight or nine repetitions should be smooth, steady, and not too difficult. They're prepping you for the real work—reps 10, 11, 12 and up. It takes a while to tire out your muscles, but after about nine reps, they're really working. That's when you'll feel the discomfort—the ache—and want to stop. Keep going! Sweating over those last few reps builds muscles!

6. Do the exercises in the order described below—legs, chest, shoulders, back, arms. The arms are last because you need them to help you do the other exercises.

7. Your muscles will tell you when they're ready to go on—listen to them. If you work up to doing the recommended number of repetitions without sweating over the last few, it's time to increase your weights. We recommend that you invest in weight accessories—small, hook-on weights of 2½, 5, or 7 pounds—which allow you to *gradually* and *safely* increase your weight.

There are no set rules about increasing weight. Use your own judgment and common sense. Don't overdo it: lifting too much weight can cause injury. But in your efforts to be cautious, don't shortchange yourself, either. You might be able to lift more than you think. Challenge yourself. You might be able to increase your weight every two weeks, even if it's only by 2½ pounds.

8. When you are ready to go on, should you increase weights or increase reps? If you want to condition, shape, and define muscles, increase the number of reps. (But don't do more reps than the maximum amount advised for each exercise.) If you're interested in big muscles, increase the weights.

REMEMBER YOUR WARM-UPS!

THE
EXERCISES

Once you've done your warm-ups and stretching, you're ready to begin the exercises.

You'll find that the exercises in this chapter give each part of your body a thorough workout. Doing all the exercises will put your body in supple, strong, tiptop shape.

Range of Weights

This is the range of weights you can expect to lift throughout training. Use these guidelines when purchasing a multi-station machine. Make sure the unit you choose has weights that reflect your lifting ability and potential.

	Men	Women
20 to 40 years old	20 to 300 lbs.	10 to 200 lbs.
50 to 60 years old	20 to 260 lbs.	10 to 150 lbs.
Older than 60	20 lbs. and up	10 lbs. and up

Remember that on your first three workouts, you should do only 10 reps per set.

Beginners' Training Chart

Use these weight guidelines for your first few workouts. Build up from there. Notice that leg muscles can lift more than arm muscles.

MULTI-STATION MACHINES	Men (Pounds)	Women (Pounds)
LEGS		
Squats	100–150	45–65
Leg press	150–200	75–100
Leg curl	35–50	25–35
Leg extension	50–70	30–45
Side leg kickout	25–30	15–20
Rear leg kickout	25–30	15–20
Calf raise	45–50	30–40
CHEST		
Bench press	65–80	35–45
Pulley flies	30–40	15–20
SHOULDERS		
Press behind neck	60–75	20–30
Standing cable cross lateral raise	20–30	10–15
Front lateral raise with cable	20–30	10–15
Bent crossover cable lateral raise	40–50	15–25
BACK		
Pulley pulldowns	60–80	30–40
Bent-over cable rowing	40–50	15–20
ARMS		
Cable biceps curl	35–45	10–20
Concentrated pulley curls	40–50	15–20
Triceps pulley pushdown	45–55	15–20
Single-arm pushdown	30–40	10–20
Triceps from shoulder kickout	20–30	10–15

NAUTILUS MACHINES	Tension Level	Tension Level
Abdominal Machine	2nd or 3rd	2nd or 3rd
Lower Back Machine	2nd or 3rd	2nd or 3rd

THE MULTI-STATION MACHINE EXERCISES

LEGS

SQUATS
3 sets of 10 to 12 reps. For thighs, buttocks.

Remove the bench. Stand under the movable arm unit and set it so that you can comfortably stand under it with your shoulders resting on the bar (or pads). Place your feet about 18 inches to 2 feet apart. Start in a standing position. Keeping your back straight, bend your knees as far as you can go. Try to go into a parallel position where your knees are level with your buttocks. Once you're in the squat position, come up slowly.

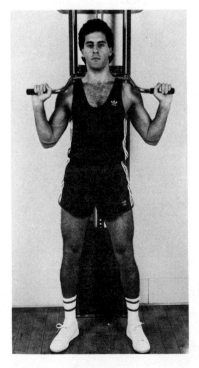
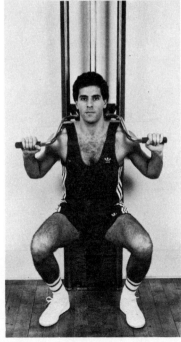

LEG PRESS
3 sets of 12 to 14 reps. For thighs, buttocks, hamstrings.

Place the bench under the arm unit. Lie on your back on the bench (or on the floor if you're not using the bench) with your feet toward the weights. Place your feet in a parallel position under each of the hand grips. Begin with legs extended in the air. Slowly bend knees to bring weight down. Bring knees down until they almost touch chest.

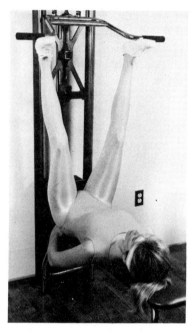 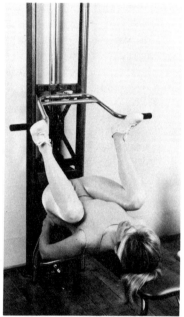

LEG CURL
3 sets of 12 to 14 reps. For hamstrings, buttocks, back leg biceps.

Lie stomach down with knees off the pad. Bring legs up slowly, feet flexed, keeping the buttocks down as you bend knees. Do not arch your back and push pelvis down into bench. Go down slowly and bring them up as soon as you're down.

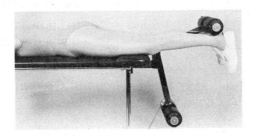

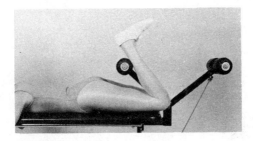

LEG EXTENSION
3 sets of 12 to 14 reps. For quadriceps.

Sit on the bench with the joint of the knees against the pad. Bring your legs up slowly, without swinging them up. Try to bring your legs up straight and have them come down without losing tension in the quads.

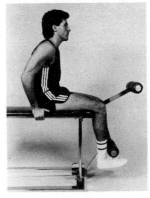 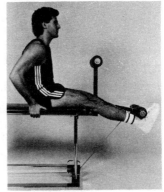

CALF PRESS
3 sets of 15 to 20 reps. (Work up to 25 per set.) For calves.

Lie on bench or floor in same position as leg press. Place your feet in a parallel position under each of the hand grips. But, this time, slide feet out under edge of grips so toes control movement of arm unit. Start with legs extended. Move arm unit down and up by pointing the toes.

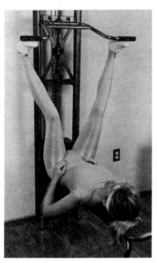 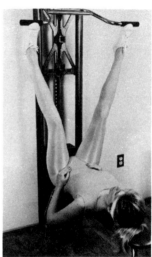

SIDE LEG KICKOUT
3 sets of 12 to 14 reps. For buttocks, outer thigh, hip.

Use low cable and foot stirrup. Stand about one foot away from, and perpendicular to, the machine. You might want to hold on to the machine with the hand that's closest. Pick up outer leg and slowly lift it up and out as far as you can. Repeat with other leg.

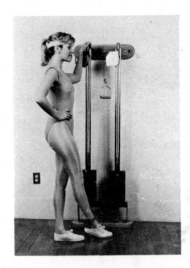 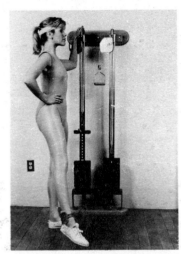

REAR LEG KICKOUT
3 sets of 12 to 14 reps. For buttocks, hamstrings.

Same as side leg kickout. Use low cable and foot stirrup. Stand about one foot away from machine, facing it. Hold on to machine. Pick up leg and slowly lift it straight back as far as you can go. Repeat with other leg.

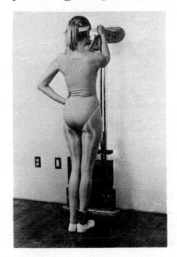 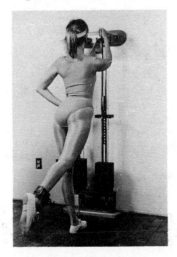

CHEST

BENCH PRESS
3 sets of 10 to 12 reps. For pectorals.

Use bench under arm unit. Lie on the bench with your eyes under the bench bar. Place your hands on the bar grips. Begin with your arms extended in the air, elbows slightly bent. Bring the arm unit down slowly and steadily until the bar is almost resting on your chest. Push it up again.

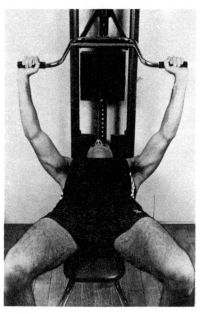 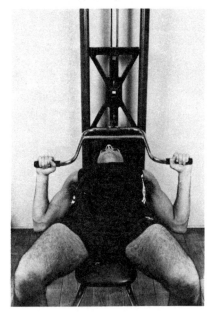

PULLEY FLIES
3 sets of 12 to 14 reps. For pectorals.

Use upper pulleys. Stand with your back to the machine about 1 1/2 feet away. Reach back, one arm at a time, to grasp pulley handles. Pull the handles out on either side of your body. Moving both arms at the same time, bring one over the other in a downward motion. Your arms will cross as they pass. Contract the pectorals as hard as you can.

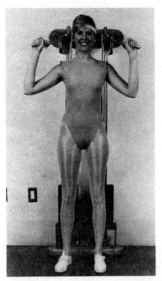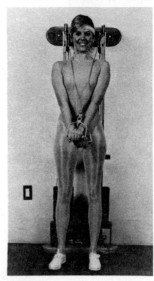

SHOULDERS

PRESS BEHIND NECK
3 sets of 10 to 12 reps. For deltoids, triceps.

Can be done sitting or standing. Sit on bench or remove it and stand. From a seated position, sit under bench press unit (you can either face the machine or sit with your back to it) and extend arms so that hands are grasping handles. Bring the bar down slowly. Rest the bar on shoulders for a second before pushing it back up.

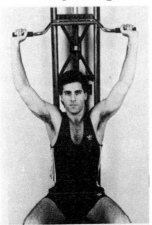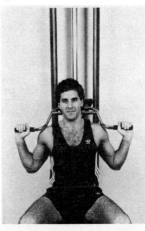

STANDING CABLE CROSS LATERAL RAISE
3 sets of 12 to 14 reps. For side deltoid.

Use bottom pulley. Stand perpendicular to machine with outer arm holding pulley handle. Pull from the bottom of the machine across the chest and up to about four inches above height of shoulder. Repeat other arm.

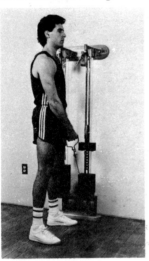 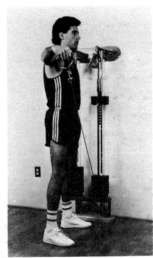

FRONT LATERAL RAISE WITH CABLE
3 sets of 12 to 14 reps. For front deltoids.

Use bottom pulley. Stand one to 1½ feet away from the machine, with your back to it. Grasp the handle at the side of your thigh. Bring arm straight up and at an angle toward the body. Repeat other arm.

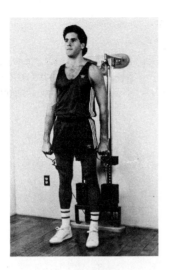 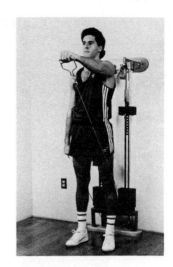

BENT CROSS-OVER CABLE LATERAL RAISE
3 sets of 12 to 14 reps. For rear deltoid.

Use bottom pulley. Bend over, pelvis back. Take a straddle position perpendicular to the machine. Outside arm grabs bottom pulley. Pull the pulley handle straight out from the machine across your body. Keep wrist slightly bent. Repeat other side.

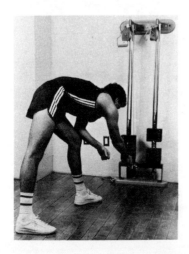 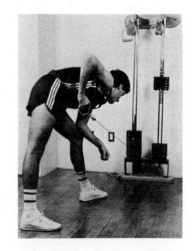

BACK

PULLEY PULLDOWNS
3 sets of 14 to 16 reps. For latissimus dorsi.

Take a kneeling or sitting position. Reach up and clasp bar at either end to get maximum amount of stretch. Pull the bar down behind the head, being careful not to hit your head. Bring it to the top of the shoulder blades and then release it slowly and evenly.

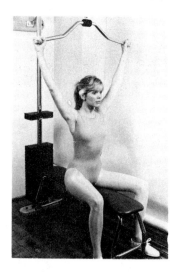 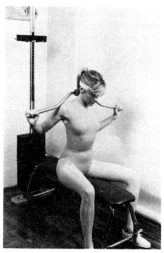

BENT-OVER CABLE ROWING
3 sets of 10 to 12 reps. (Work up to 14 reps.) For latissimus dorsi.

Use bottom pulley. Face machine and take a running stance. Rest one arm on front knee for support. Begin with the handle down and bring it up to the waist in a sawing motion, lifting the elbow in the air. Repeat with other arm.

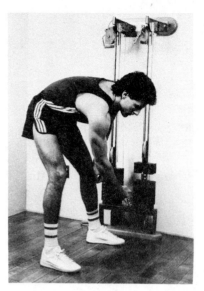 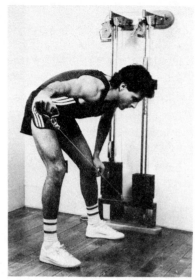

ARMS

CABLE BICEPS CURLS
3 sets of 10 to 12 reps. (Work up to 14 reps.) For forearms and biceps.

Use bottom pulleys. Either face the machine or stand with your back to it. Grasp both bottom pulleys, arms extended down, inner forearms facing machine, wrists slightly bent in. Exercise can be done with both arms at the same time or alternating them. Keeping elbows in place, bring hand up to shoulder level. Lean the body back slightly.

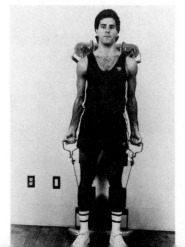 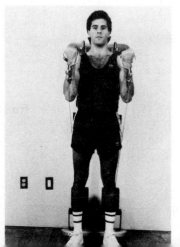

CONCENTRATED PULLEY CURLS
3 sets of 12 to 14 reps. For biceps.

Use bottom pulley. Squat in front of the pulley, facing, or perpendicular to, the machine. Rest one arm on same side quad. Begin with inner forearm of working arm facing downward. Bring handle up no farther than waist level. The small distance traveled concentrates the curl movement at the peak of the biceps.

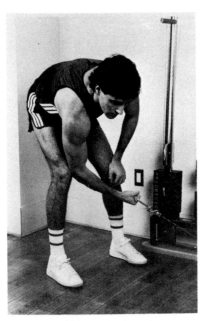
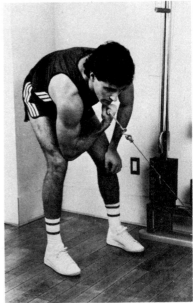

TRICEPS PULLEY PUSHDOWN
3 sets of 14 to 18 reps. (Work up to 20 reps.) For triceps.

Take a standing position in front of the pulldown unit. Each hand grasps bar in the middle, holding it at chest level. Begin by pushing bar down slowly so that arms are extended. Bring bar up steadily. During down and up movements, keep elbows tucked in.

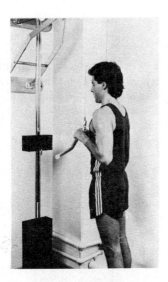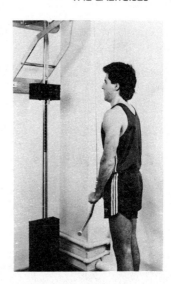

SINGLE-ARM PULLEY PUSHDOWN
3 sets of 12 to 14 reps. (Work up to 16 or 18 reps.) For triceps.

Similar to triceps pulldown. Use top cable. Hold handle at chest level. Keep elbow tucked in. Bring arm down as far as it will go; bring up steadily.

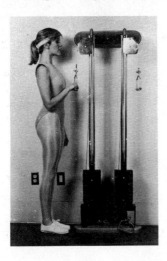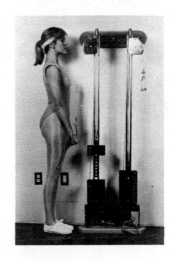

TRICEPS FROM SHOULDER KICKOUT
3 sets of 10 to 12 reps. For triceps.

Use top pulleys. Stand with your back to machine. Steady arm with other hand under elbow. Take pulley and hold it near your ear. Pull; forearm moves straight out.

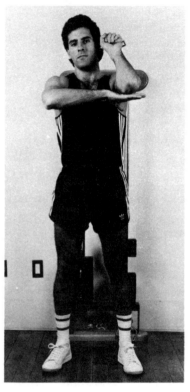 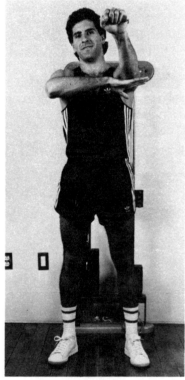

THE NAUTILUS EXERCISES

The following exercises can only be performed on Nautilus home exercise machines.

THE LOWER BACK MACHINE
Start with 20 to 25 reps. (Work up to 40 reps.) For lumbar region of back and sides.

Strap yourself in. Place your feet toward the back end of the foot rest so that your legs are extended and it looks like you're standing in the machine. Cross arms over your chest. Position yourself against the pads, keeping your back straight. Push back against the pads, breathing out. Don't arch. Return to the starting position. Bend forward a little more.

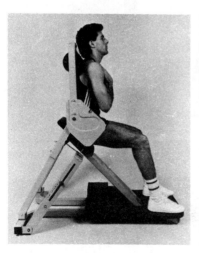
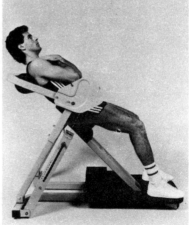

THE ABDOMINAL MACHINE
Start with 20 to 25 reps. (Work up to 40 reps.) For abdominal muscles.

Adjust seat so that you're sitting comfortably: knees slightly bent and feet flat on the floor. Sit on the set, knees wide apart. Adjust seat so that the chest pads are at chest level. To begin, bend forward as far as you can, breathing out, tensing the abdominals. The back should be curved—not flat—as you go over. Hold the bottom position for a second and come back up. Contract your stomach muscles and come back up slowly, resisting the temptation to fly back up. The slower you go coming down the more negative resistance is working on your muscles.

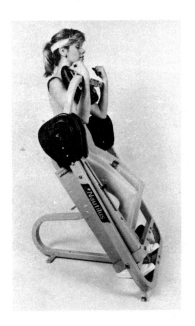
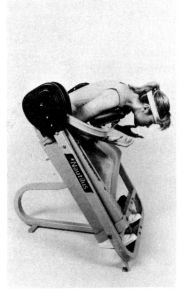

REMEMBER YOUR COOL-DOWNS!

Doing More

There are several variations on the basic weight-training program that will take you to higher levels of development.

• Increase your repetitions. Follow our guidelines and try doing the highest number of reps recommended for each exercise.

• Add one more set to your workout. Instead of doing three sets, do four and continue to increase weights as you improve.

• Try circuit training, using every station or every machine in sequence without stopping in between. To do this, you must set up the stations so that they are ready for you when you get there—so you can go from one to another without stopping to adjust the equipment. If your machine has only one weight stack, learn how to move the selector pin speedily so you can go from one exercise to the next smoothly. Vary your circuit training routine: Try going to all the stations three or four times nonstop. Or, mix aerobic exercise into your weight-training sequence. Jog in place, bicycle, or jump rope for 30 seconds in between each station. You'll really work up a sweat and get your muscles going that way!

BUYER'S GUIDE TO WEIGHT-TRAINING MACHINES

Machines at a Glance

Compact, solid, durable

Marcy Bodybar	$250
Excel's Brutus Bodytech	$700

Good for beginners

DP Gympac	$485
Billard Family Fitness Center	$200
Soloflex	$565

Large, multi-station for several users at once

Paramount Fitness Trainer	$3,200
Paramount Fitness Trainer II	$2,700
Marcy Family Fitness Center	$1,250
Universal Power-Pak 300	$1,983
Universal Power-Pak 400	$3,153
Weider	$10,000

Total Gym from Westbend
    The Competition Plus $395
    The Pro $495
    The Pro Plus $499

The Nautilus Machines
    Nautilus Abdominal Machine $485
    Nautilus Lower Back Machine $485

Size and Cost

Before you buy your weight-training machine, there are two points to keep in mind—size and cost. What kind of home gym are you setting up? Will it fill up a large room or fill up an unused corner in a busy room? How much do you want to spend?

Luckily, one of the advantages of multi-station machines is that they can be as elaborate or as simple as you please—without sacrificing any aspect of the basic workout.

If you have a whole room set aside for your home gym, make sure you have space around the machine. You'll need space around the leg exercise units and extra area around the machine for circuit training or for stretching out. If you don't have much space to spare, look into one of the machines designed for easy storage. A wall-mounted exerciser can be set up easily behind a door or in an out-of-the-way corner.

Construction

Because there are so many pieces of machinery on the market, it's a good idea to carefully check out any piece that you're considering buying. First of all, how is it made? Does the material look like cardboard or is it strong enough to endure constant use? Second, how is the machine held together? Look for machines that are welded or soldered together. Equipment put together with nuts and bolts won't last as long with heavy use over time. A strong, well-constructed machine is also an important safety factor.

Weight Capacity

Machines come with different capabilities. Check out a machine's potential. You don't want to outgrow it in a short time. For example, if a machine comes with 100 pounds of weight and you're determined to test your limits, you might want 150 more pounds as an option.

Just as you don't want to have too little weight, neither do you want too much. Remember to take into consideration the weight of the apparatus itself. Sometimes you don't even need to start off with a weight; lifting the weight of the bar could be a workout in itself. Check to see what the minimum is on each machine. Increments of 10 pounds are the norm, but some machines start with 25 to 50 pounds. Using the weight guidelines on pages 23-24 and knowing your athletic aptitude, take weight count into consideration when making a purchase.

The following list of machines is a sampling of what's on the market. We've advised you of the companies who make superb equipment and given you a smattering of the two- and three-star varieties. Remember, many of the companies mentioned here make more than one piece of equipment. Most of the equipment listed can be found at sporting goods stores around the country. Or contact the manufacturer for a distributor in your area.

Paramount Fitness Trainer
Price: $3,200
2 weight stacks of 210 and 105 pounds.
Optional stacks of 310 and 155 pounds also available.

Paramount has an excellent reputation. Its flashy, chrome equipment is also strong and well built. The standard unit comes with chest/shoulder press and bench, high pulley with lat bar, low pulley with t-bar, stirrups, and ankle straps. A solid guide rod selects the weights. The unit can be expanded to include a knee raise, leg extension, leg curl, leg press, and squat option. The chest station contains 210 pounds, the high and low pulley systems have 105 pounds. Weights are black; chrome is also available.

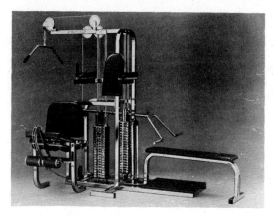

Paramount Fitness Trainer II
Price: $2,700
One weight stack of 170 pounds.
Optional 210 pounds also available.

The Trainer II resembles the Trainer in standard functions and options to expand. One weight stack is used at all stations.

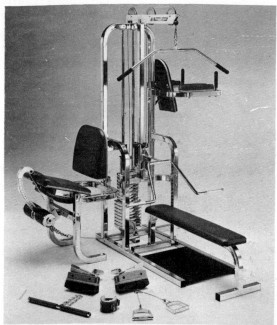

Marcy Bodybar 2000

Price: $250
One stack of 100 pounds.
Optional weights up to 180 pounds also available.

Marcy always gets rave reviews from people in the know about weight-training equipment. It's got the qualities expert bodybuilders look for in a piece of equipment: strong, solid, and well built with heavy-duty construction.

For its price, the Bodybar 2000 is a bargain. It offers a complete workout in a small space for a small price. Its slim design makes it useful in the smallest of home gyms. Despite its small stature, the Bodybar can make strong muscles. It uses the most highly recommended weight plates—made of cast iron, not covered cement or vinyl. Its compact design includes high and low pulley system, eight-position lifting arm, bench press, and a leg curl/leg extension unit. The Bodybar 2000 is a wall-mount unit. An optional platform can be purchased as an accessory ($98) to make the unit freestanding. The gym can be expanded with other accessories.

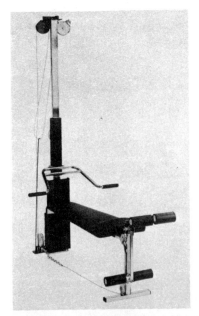

Marcy Family Fitness Center
Price: $1,250
Three stacks of 100, 180 and 220 pounds.
Optional weights up to 320 pounds also available.

Again, Marcy's heavy-duty construction and reliable name can be counted on for a quality product. The Family Fitness Center is an expanded version of the Bodybar. It has four separate stations, so four people can work out on it at the same time. There are three sets of weights: 220 pounds at the bench press, two 50-pound stacks at the high and low pulley systems, 180 pounds at the lat machine. An abdominal board is also included.

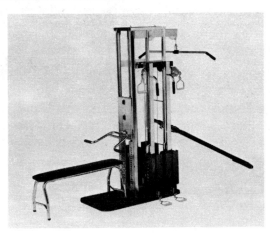

Universal Power-Pak 300
Price: $1,983
One weight stack of 100 pounds.
Optional 180 and 260 pounds also available.

Universal was in the limelight for years as the only company with a multi-unit station. If a commercial gym or health spa owned a machine, chances are it was a Universal. When other companies got into the act, Universal upgraded

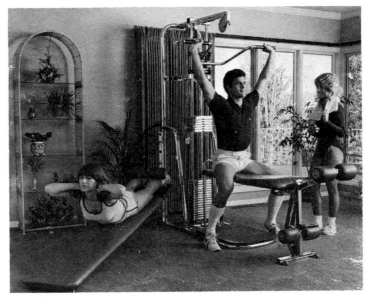

its machines. Today, Universal's home gyms are as sturdy and safe as those designed for commercial use. The home machines are made of steel tubing and finished in nickel chrome.

The Power-Pak 300 has a chest station, high and low pulleys, and accessories for low pulley work. Optional chrome weights are available. One special feature of Universal equipment is the nylon alloy bushings around the weights for smooth strokes as the weights travel up and down the shaft.

Universal Power-Pak 400
Price: $3,153
Two weight stacks of 115 and 100 pounds.
Optional weights of 180 and 260 pounds also available.

The Power-Pak 400's design is similar to the 300, except that it's larger and can work up to three people at a time. It has the same standard features as the 300, but has two sets of weights: 5 to 115 pounds for the pulley system and 100 for

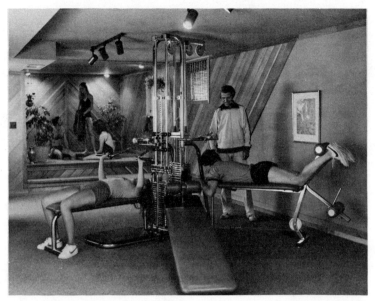

the chest station. Accessories to expand the unit's capabilities are also available.

DP Gympac 1500
Price: $485
One weight stack of 110 pounds.
Optional weights of up to 88 pounds also available.

DP makes fitness products for all sports; it manufactures everything from vitamins and basketballs to golf carts and Ping-Pong balls. So when it comes to weight-training equipment, DP isn't exactly considered a specialist in the field.

The DP 1500 is recommended as a good piece of equipment for a beginner. Because it's held together with nuts and bolts, it's not designed for very heavy use. In fact, more time has been spent on the 1500's storage design than on its usefulness. The unit has a removable bench that can be folded up on its wall mounting or rolled away on its rubber

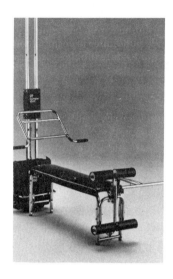

tires. Because it includes all the vital parts—bench, pulleys, and leg extension/leg curl—you will get every part of the basic workout.

Weider Circuit 12 Flex Tech Fitness Center
Price: $10,000
Seven weight stacks with 10 to 657 pounds.
Optional weights up to 587 pounds also available.

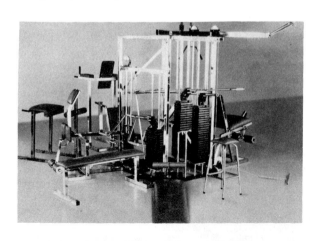

Weider is another well-known name in the fitness industry, featuring bodybuilding equipment from barbells to training clothes and nutritional supplements. The Weider Circuit 12 Flex Tech Fitness Center has seven separate weight stacks. Besides the regular bodybuilding features like shoulder and bench press, leg curl/leg extension, pulley systems, and lat pulldown, it also has leg press, chinning bar, Roman chair, and dipping bar.

Excel's Brutus Bodytech
Price: $700
One weight stack of 100 pounds.
Optional weights of 340 pounds also available.

Excel has made its name in solid benches. The Brutus Bodytech looks like its name—strong, heavy duty—and is equipped with leg curl/leg extension and lat pulldown. Don't let the simplicity of the Bodytech's design fool you: this is one of the stronger, more durable machines. It is recommended for beginners and intermediates interested in lifting up to 340 pounds. With a freestanding stand, price is $100 more.

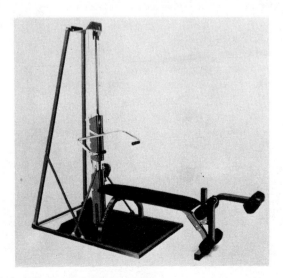

Billard Family Fitness Center
Price: $200
One stack of 120 pounds.

Billard is an excellent manufacturer of free-weight equipment—benches, barbells, and dumbbells. The Family Fitness Center is not as sturdy as other units, but it is a good beginning piece of equipment. It is designed to be wall mounted and is equipped with bench press and leg curl/leg extension unit. The bench has collapsible legs for easy storage. Without taking up too much floor space, it can be stored against the wall. An optional support piece to make it free-standing is also available. Billard equipment is available only through retail outlets.

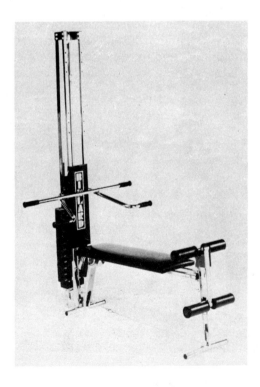

Soloflex
Price: $565
Weights up to 300 pounds

Soloflex's simple, bold design and heavy-duty construction make it an elegant addition to any home gym. Constructed of steel and stainless steel with a hardwood platform, its unique weight-resistance system uses rubber weightstraps that are attached in such a way that as you lift, you pull the rubber weight, giving your muscles a variable-resistance workout. Soloflex offers multiple-station work: the board triples as a bench press, abdominal board, and platform for back work.

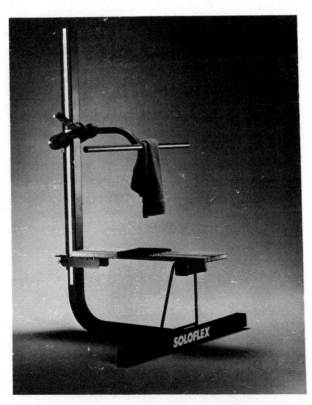

Total Gym from Westbend

The Total Gym—either the Competition Plus, the Pro, or the Pro Plus—is an innovation in the evolution of weight-training equipment. Unlike most other "weight" training apparatus, the Total Gym uses the person's own body weight as resistance instead of weights. It's simple in design with only an abdominal board and two arm pulleys. You increase or decrease the workload by changing the height of the glideboard. The steeper the incline, the more challenging the exercise.

Total Gym comes with its own set of instructions. You can get an aerobic workout or strengthen or tone specific body parts. You can also get in shape for specific sports—warming up the arm muscles for tennis or swimming, for example, or the legs for running.

The Competition Plus
Price: $395

The Competition Plus has a welded frame and is constructed of heavy-gauge steel. It has seven resistance levels to choose from and is 38 inches when folded for storage.

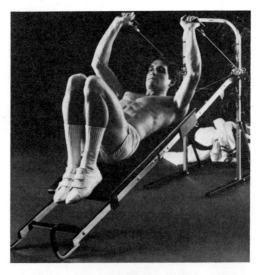

The Pro
Price: $495

The Pro is designed similarly to the Competition Plus, but has nine resistance levels for a tougher workout. (The higher the board, the harder the exercise.) It features a heavy-gauge steel tube frame. It measures 48 inches when stored.

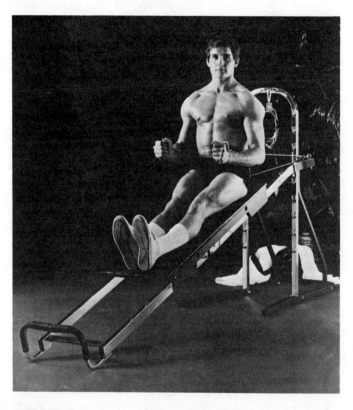

The Pro Plus
Price: $499

The Pro Plus offers the best workout with 11 resistance levels, allowing for a very steep position. The Pro Plus comes with a squat stand to facilitate leg exercises. It is only 48

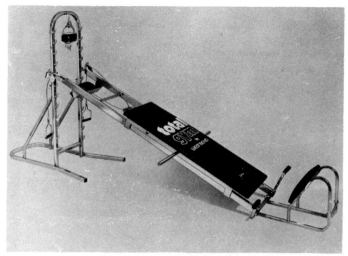

inches when stored and has a built-in weight frame that can support additional weights for optional exercises.

Nautilus Abdominal Machine
Price: $485
Measures 48 × 38 × 35½ inches

This space-age-looking equipment is easier to use than it looks. The abdominal machine isolates stomach muscles for a trim, strong, flexible waist. Its frame is made of heavy tubular steel and it's cushioned with tough Naugahyde. Nine graduated tensions make your workout tougher as you improve. You can assemble the machine yourself in only a few minutes.

Nautilus Lower Back Machine
Price: $485
Measures 54 × 51 × 35 inches

Nautilus first developed a lower back machine for its home gym series because, according to research, about 80 to 90 percent of all Americans have problems with their lower backs. This machine is used for rehabilitation, prevention, and cure of back problems. Like the abdominal machine, it is made of tubular steel and is cushioned in Naugahyde. It also features nine graduated tensions.

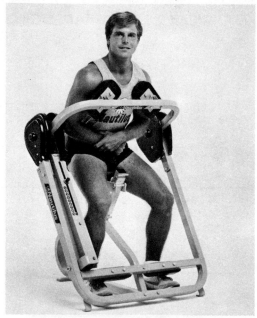

Nautilus Abdominal Machine

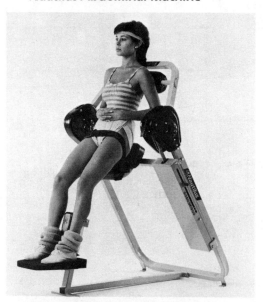

Nautilus Lower Back Machine

THE 12-WEEK WEIGHT-TRAINING LOG

	Week 1			Week 2			Week 3		
	Day 1	Day 2	Day 3	Day 1	Day 2	Day 3	Day 1	Day 2	Day 3
Time of day									
Mood									
Exercises—Rep/Weights									
Squats	8/40			8/40			8/40		
Leg press									
Leg curl									
Leg extension									
Side leg kickout									
Rear leg kickout									
Calf press									
Bench press									
Pulley flies									
Press behind neck									
Standing cable cross lateral raise									
Front lateral raise with cable									
Bent cross-over cable lateral raise									
Pulley pulldowns									
Bent-over cable rowing									
Cable biceps curls									
Concentrated pulley curls									
Triceps pulley pushdown									
Single-arm pulley pushdown									
Triceps from shoulder kickout									
Nautilus lower back machine									
Nautilus abdominal machine									

	Week 4			Week 5			Week 6		
	Day 1	Day 2	Day 3	Day 1	Day 2	Day 3	Day 1	Day 2	Day 3
Time of day									
Mood									
Exercises—Rep/Weights									
Squats	8/40			8/40			8/40		
Leg press									
Leg curl									
Leg extension									
Side leg kickout									
Rear leg kickout									
Calf press									
Bench press									
Pulley flies									
Press behind neck									
Standing cable cross lateral raise									
Front lateral raise with cable									
Bent cross-over cable lateral raise									
Pulley pulldowns									
Bent-over cable rowing									
Cable biceps curls									
Concentrated pulley curls									
Triceps pulley pushdown									
Single-arm pulley pushdown									
Triceps from shoulder kickout									
Nautilus lower back machine									
Nautilus abdominal machine									

	Week 7			Week 8			Week 9		
	Day 1	Day 2	Day 3	Day 1	Day 2	Day 3	Day 1	Day 2	Day 3
Time of day									
Mood									
Exercises—Rep/Weights									
Squats	8/40			8/40			8/40		
Leg press									
Leg curl									
Leg extension									
Side leg kickout									
Rear leg kickout									
Calf press									
Bench press									
Pulley flies									
Press behind neck									
Standing cable cross lateral raise									
Front lateral raise with cable									
Bent cross-over cable lateral raise									
Pulley pulldowns									
Bent-over cable rowing									
Cable biceps curls									
Concentrated pulley curls									
Triceps pulley pushdown									
Single-arm pulley pushdown									
Triceps from shoulder kickout									
Nautilus lower back machine									
Nautilus abdominal machine									

	Week 10			Week 11			Week 12		
	Day 1	Day 2	Day 3	Day 1	Day 2	Day 3	Day 1	Day 2	Day 3
Time of day									
Mood									
Exercises—Rep/Weights									
Squats	8/40			8/40			8/40		
Leg press									
Leg curl									
Leg extension									
Side leg kickout									
Rear leg kickout									
Calf press									
Bench press									
Pulley flies									
Press behind neck									
Standing cable cross lateral raise									
Front lateral raise with cable									
Bent cross-over cable lateral raise									
Pulley pulldowns									
Bent-over cable rowing									
Cable biceps curls									
Concentrated pulley curls									
Triceps pulley pushdown									
Single-arm pulley pushdown									
Triceps from shoulder kickout									
Nautilus lower back machine									
Nautilus abdominal machine									

VILLARD'S AT-HOME GYM SERIES

( ) 72971-4 **ROWING**
              by Michael T. Cannell $2.95; in Canada, $4.25

( ) 72972-2 **FREE WEIGHTS**
              by Judith Zimmer $2.95; in Canada, $4.25

( ) 72973-0 **STATIONARY BICYCLES**
              by Michael T. Cannell $2.95; in Canada $4.25

( ) 72974-9 **WEIGHT MACHINES**
              by Judith Zimmer $2.95; in Canada, $4.25

Buy these books at your local bookstore or use this handy coupon for ordering.

Villard Books, Dept. 14-1, 201 East 50th Street, New York, New York 10022

Please send me the books I have checked above.
I am enclosing $ _____.*
For each title, please add 95¢ for postage and handling. Send check or money order—no cash or C.O.D.s, please. Make check payable to Villard Books.

Name_____
                           (please print)

Address _____

City/State _____ Zip _____

Please allow 4-6 weeks for delivery. This offer expires 12/31/85.

*Residents of NY, IL, WI, MD please add sales tax.